The Procrastinator's Guide to Killing Yourself

Living when life feels unliveable

GARETH EDWARDS

CONTENTS

YOUR JOURNEY, YOUR WAY

This book is a guide,
but you must always walk your own path.

It is how I found a way forward
rather than a way out.

It is not advice about what you should do.

It is my journey of 'living myself'.

I hope it helps your own.

Love, Gareth

WHO IS THIS BOOK FOR?

This book is for those of us who are looking into a huge black hole and feeling that life is not worth living.

So that's probably all of us at some point in our life.

But for some of us, that feeling keeps coming up and the path we are on comes to a dead-end of circling thoughts, feelings and behaviours that seem to try to answer the question 'should I kill myself?'

If you are staring into the abyss in the cul de sac of your soul, this book is for you.

This book might also help those of us who love someone who is trying to answer the question 'should I kill myself?'

So that's probably all of us at some point in our life too.

The pain of having a loved-one in pain and feeling unable to ease that pain is doubly painful.

Actually it's more like pain squared:

$$\text{pain} \times \text{pain} = p^p$$

If you are supporting someone to step away from the abyss, this book is for you.

The purpose of this book is to show you how I found a way forward rather than a way out.

We all find our own way.

LET'S STOP TALKING ABOUT SUICIDE

I choose to avoid using the word 'suicide'.

It was coined to criminalise and pass moral judgment on a profound and legitimate human experience.

I believe that wanting to kill yourself is part of what makes you human.

I do not believe that wanting to kill yourself means you are sick or a bad person.

I write about wanting to kill myself as something that happened in my past, as it is less strong than it was during my teens and twenties.

I still have thoughts and feelings about killing myself and occasionally I have the urge to act on those thoughts and feelings.

The difference now is that I have discovered and learnt different ideas and techniques to feel more comfort with these types of experiences.

Rather than feeling worried when the question 'should I kill myself?' returns, it instead fascinates me and has become an opportunity to enrich my life with renewed meaning and purpose.

THE DAY I DECIDED TO LIVE, AGAIN

I'm standing alone in the centre of the living room.

My friend is bustling around the other rooms while my social worker tells me about the rent and the impact on my sickness benefits.

I hear them both but I'm mostly listening to my inner voice calmly and confidently say, "We will die here".

"Here we go again" I think.

I manage to smile through my despair.

My social worker takes this as a sign that I like the flat that she's found for me, just a few months after being discharged from the local psychiatric ward.

GARETH EDWARDS

But I'm smiling for a different reason.

I'm smiling because, after more than a year of fighting this inner voice, I think I might have found a use for it.

I'm still many years away from welcoming and celebrating it, but at least I'm less terrified and traumatised by it.

"So what do you think Gareth?" she says with a hopeful look in her eye.

My friend pops his head out of the bedroom and gives me an equally hopeful smile as if to say 'it'll be alright mate'.

"I'll think about it," I mumble.

The inner voice gives way to an inner vision.

I see myself sat in this living room, smoking endless hand-rolled cigarettes, hiding from the world except for visits to the psychiatric outpatient clinic and the benefits office.

I see worried phone calls and visits from family and friends; lovingly trying to coax me back to the person I was before all this began.

THE PROCRASTINATOR'S GUIDE TO KILLING YOURSELF

I see repeating readmissions to the psychiatric inpatient ward, a constant calibrating of medication and getting to know my nurses better than my friends.

But mostly I see myself dead in the room I am standing in right now.

And I smile again, because I have already had this experience many times and have found ways to step beyond it, and even step up from it.

Wanting to kill myself is the flipside of the coin of wanting to 'live myself.'

In the old days, before camera phones and social media, you would take a roll of plastic film with tiny, dark images to the chemists to be made in to large, fully coloured pictures.

The film was called 'the negatives' and it was taken into a laboratory called a dark room to be developed into photographs.

My despair, distress and desperation are like the small, inverse feelings of the large and colourful life I want to live.

The desire to kill myself is really the desire to 'live myself' but feeling it is impossible.

In the dark room of my own learning I've found that if I can be aware of my feelings of wanting to kill myself, and accept them without judging them as good or bad, then the pain is reduced, and I can reconnect with my desire to live the life I want to live.

The positive only exists in relation to the negative.

Like day needs night, black needs white and shade needs light. The life that feels impossible begins to feel possible.

I leave the flat knowing I will never return.

I decide, again, to live.

THE PROCRASTINATOR'S GUIDE TO KILLING YOURSELF

So you want to kill yourself.

Feel like you can't go on anymore and you just want to end it all?

That life has become ... unliveable?

Me too.

But not today.

And not as often as I used to.

But it feels like it wasn't so long ago I felt that way every day.

Every damn day, as the saying goes.

I had days where my only goal was to find a reason to live. Just one reason. There were days, many damn days, where even that was beyond me and I clung to life with a force I still struggle to comprehend.

So what right?

I still have no idea what you are going through.

True.

I only know what I've gone through. And the ideas and techniques I've stumbled across, made my own and now use to help me stay alive.

The most useful of these for me, when it is literally a matter of life and death, is procrastination. Delaying the act of killing myself is more helpful than fighting the feeling of wanting to kill myself.

Because let me tell you something that you probably already know.

Something I think we all know and that most of us would rather not know.

I think everybody thinks about killing themselves.

THE PROCRASTINATOR'S GUIDE TO KILLING YOURSELF

Everybody.

It is an important part of being human, of experiencing times of deep distress and recognising the impermanence of life. At some point in all our lives we will arrive at a place where we can only see a way out rather than a way forward.

People have had these challenging and distressing experiences for as long as there have been people.

Whatever your stance on the question 'why are we here?' these dark and difficult experiences either supported our survival as we evolved or are part of a grand design.

So we have these experiences for a reason.

And I believe it is because they have meaning.

Sure they can be painful and scary for us, as well as our loved ones and society in general. But my experience is that the more we hide painful and scary things with shame, stigma and taboo the more powerful they become.

Darkness within us and in society must be met with more light, not less.

GARETH EDWARDS

For some, the idea of killing our self is a fleeting thought that, whilst alarming, is straightforward to disarm and passes quickly. For others, the idea lingers and nags away at us until it is the only thought.

And it is in these situations that I have found it best to flip traditional wisdom and 'do put off until tomorrow what I could do today'.

Thinking about whether my life was worth living was not a sign that it should end. It was a sign that I needed a different way of thinking.

I wanted to kill myself more than I wanted to carry on living.

Accepting that took the pressure off working out why I wanted to kill myself.

Rather than hating myself for hating myself I said 'I will kill myself, just not now'. The 'not now' started very small. Literally putting it off for a moment.

And the moments became minutes, then hours and eventually a whole day. Then days followed each other and became a week, a month and a year.

A lifetime.

THE PROCRASTINATOR'S GUIDE TO KILLING YOURSELF

Even within those early moments of delay, a space began to open up for me as I stopped ruminating on whether to do it or not. The decision had been made and postponed, like a meeting no one really wants to attend.

And in that space something new began to grow.

It was still too early to call it hope, though I believe it established the ground from which that gentle flower could blossom. It was more like respite.

Like when you take your shoes off after a long day. You know you will put them on again in the future, but for now you can stretch out your squashed up feet and enjoy the cool air on your toes.

So sure, I can relate to the feeling that you want to kill yourself.

I think it is an important part of who you are, of who we all are, as human beings.

But before you act on that decision, kick of your shoes for a little while and feel the breeze.

You might find life returns.

THE NIGHT I DECIDED TO LIVE

Statistics kept me alive when I most wanted to kill myself.

In the midst of my despair I knew two things.

The first was that the country was gripped by a 'suicide crisis' of young men killing themselves before their 25th birthday. The second was that I was not going to be one of them.

Don't misunderstand me; I wanted to kill myself.

It just felt… insulting to have my death chalked up as another data point.

So I waited.

THE PROCRASTINATOR'S GUIDE TO KILLING YOURSELF

I allowed the daily desperation to wash through me like a sieve.

Every waking moment was like being in a courtroom with the case for and against killing myself going back and forth.

Sleep was worse, full of vivid visions and waking up frequently, screaming silently.

My life had ground to a halt and the few conversations I had with people were twisted into compelling reasons to kill myself now.

Every newspaper headline, film, book and TV show became part of a global hopelessness I felt in the core of my being.

Footbridges became terrifying ordeals, with lengthy pauses by the handrail, every fibre of my being screaming 'jump'!

The radio taunted me with the Lenny Kravitz song Fly Away urging me on:

"I wish that I could fly, into the sky, I want to get away, I want to fly away"

GARETH EDWARDS

As the clock clicked over to 12.01am on my 25th birthday I smiled for the first time in a long time.

I had made it.

Now, time to die.

I lay on my bed and stared at the window.

The curtain covered one of the four glass panes with the other three gathering condensation in the cold winter night.

And then I saw it, spelt out like a message from the other side.

G-A-Z

My nickname - Gaz.

Right there, etched into the condensation on the window, calling me, telling me that here was the way, an end to the torment.

Just step through and jump. Fly away.

Paralysed by fear I did something I had not done before. I stopped fighting.

THE PROCRASTINATOR'S GUIDE TO KILLING YOURSELF

I accepted that I really, really wanted to open that window and jump off the roof. The panic eased a little and I began to run through what I would do in my mind.

I saw myself get up from my bed, walk over to the desk and clear a space so I could stand on it. Climbing up, I would open the right-hand window with the A and Z of GAZ written on them, and clamber through.

I imagined what it would be like to be stood on the steep, tiled roof in the middle of the night in the middle of winter and how I would have to hold on tightly to the window frame so I could pick my time to jump rather than just fall.

I closed my eyes and thought about what I would think about up there on the roof in the moments before I let go of that window frame.

Of how peaceful it would be to know that this living nightmare would be over. And how that brief freedom of flight might feel in my final moments.

Then something unusual happened.

I laughed.

It was just a little laugh, more like a dry cough, but it was enough to shake me from my mental rehearsal.

What I had found funny, in a dark and morbid way, was that I had got to the part of killing myself where I did not actually die.

My attic bedroom was only on the third floor of my house. At worst I would probably break a leg, or even more embarrassingly, just sprain an ankle.

The image of me sprawled out in our backyard, squirming in pain, while my best friend stuck his head out the window to ask me, in his lovingly Northern English way 'what are you up to Gaz?' was so ridiculous to me that I laughed.

And in that moment I knew two new things.

The first was that I still had enough of myself left to be able to laugh at myself.

The second was that I was not going to kill myself.

LIVING WHEN LIFE FEELS UNLIVEABLE

Let's say you are successfully procrastinating about killing yourself – what now?

Well first of all, take a little time and space to celebrate that!

Every moment not spent on the why, when, where and how of killing yourself is a moment that can be used answering the question of how to live yourself.

But how do you do that? How do you live when life feels unliveable?

The truthful answer is – I do not know.

The next bit of the truthful answer is – you do know.

And the final bit of the truthful answer is - I know how I lived when life felt unliveable.

So that is what I have for you.

The way I did it.

I have described them as steps, as most of us like a sense of order. But I see them as more of an upward moving spiral than a strict sequence.

Less like a ladder and more like a staircase in a medieval castle. As we slowly ascend, we revisit steps in a similar position but one rung higher.

It is the same with these steps.

As we sweep past familiar looking thoughts, feelings and behaviours it is with a higher level of appreciation and understanding.

This allows us to learn something new, mix it with what we already knew to be true and then think, feel or do something different.

So we can say 'yes I knew that already, and now I know it more so' or 'yes I felt that already, and now I feel it more so'.

THE PROCRASTINATOR'S GUIDE TO KILLING YOURSELF

And perhaps more importantly we can say 'yes I do that already, and now I do it more so'.

I have given each step a phrase about surrendering.

This is not a word or a concept I used at the time, but it is how these steps now feel to me.

Wanting to kill ourselves is often called 'giving up' as if we are surrendering to the desire to die. For me, I am surrendering to my desire to live and I 'give up' on all the things that diminish or interfere with that desire.

Please check every step against what you feel is true for you and take only what is useful and can be blended into your own truth.

STEP 1: STAY ALIVE

SURRENDERING TO SURVIVAL

When I wanted to kill myself it felt very primal, like I was a frightened animal battling to stay alive.

Which, of course, I was.

There was no actual external threat, though I'd say living in modern society is just as scary as stumbling across the odd tiger in the jungle.

At the time it felt like I was trying to save myself from myself.

It was a matter of life and death. So my first step was to survive. I found accepting that I wanted to kill myself and delaying the act was effective for me.

THE PROCRASTINATOR'S GUIDE TO KILLING YOURSELF

Years later when I started work in a detox and rehab centre, I found 'delaying' is a well-established technique in addictions.

Rather than struggle with cravings to drink alcohol or use drugs, some people find it useful to say to themselves "I will have a drink or use drugs, but I will do it later".

It seems to take the pressure off the internal struggle of wanting to drink alcohol or use drugs and wanting to not drink alcohol or use drugs.

With the pressure reduced some people find the urge passes and by the time they get to 'later' the urge is forgotten or less intense.

I didn't know any of this at the time I was procrastinating about killing myself.

I just knew I was finished with fighting myself.

I wanted to kill myself.

I had felt that way for long enough to know it wasn't going to just pass on it's own. In fact, I felt like it would never pass, that I would feel this way forever.

GARETH EDWARDS

On the night I decided to live I had a mixture of thoughts and feelings swirling round inside me that led to this certainty I wasn't going to kill myself.

Partly it was the length of time I had been feeling this way and the thought that if I was going to kill myself, I would have done it by now. There was also a little pride that I had out-witted the statisticians by living past my 25th birthday.

I think this gave me a sense of control over my thoughts, feelings and behaviours, though at the time I probably didn't see it that way.

Rehearsing how I would kill myself was part of the procrastination and I feel this helped, as I had chosen to imagine killing myself rather than actually killing myself.

When we choose, we have control, even if we are unaware we are making a choice. Which was important, as it was this feeling of being out of control that terrified me and made me believe that killing myself was inevitable.

It felt like these thoughts, feelings and behaviours were happening to me, that I was at their mercy rather than their master.

THE PROCRASTINATOR'S GUIDE TO KILLING YOURSELF

Looking back it feels like a paradox, that to feel in control I needed to surrender.

A huge part of that was accepting an idea that has been with me for as long as I can remember and gets revisited and reframed often. I think it is something we all encounter and it starts when we are very young.

Quite soon after we start talking we start asking 'why?'

Some of us never stop.

With my son I did my best to give an answer when he asked 'why?'

And of course for every answer he would pause, look puzzled, and then look back at me and again ask 'why?'

This would carry on until I had no more answers.

But rather than say 'because', as that never worked for me as an answer when I was growing up, I would say 'I don't know'.

And to my surprise, he seemed satisfied with that.

He still had his question but he knew he wasn't going to get the answer from me.

At some point, most people stop asking 'why?' For those of us that don't, it can be a frustrating journey.

Take any belief system (scientific, religious, cultural, spiritual) and it ultimately ends up at 'we don't know'. I have found the more I can be satisfied with that; the easier life seems to become.

Because life is meaningless.

We don't know why we are here. We have a bunch of interesting ideas on 'how' we are here, like divine creation or evolution, but not 'why'.

Some people are quite happy with the answer 'because'.

I admire and even envy those people.

But it is not for me.

I still have that insatiable curiosity toddlers have, exploring my world to make sense of it. At times this leads to temper tantrums, especially when the world seems cruel or confusing.

THE PROCRASTINATOR'S GUIDE TO KILLING YOURSELF

I stamp my feet and shake my fists at the sky and shout 'why?!'

The only answer I have found so far is that the pursuit of the answer is the answer itself.

In a meaningless universe I am the meaning-maker.

It feels like a dance between despair and delight, swirling endlessly within me.

"Life is meaningless, so what's the point?"' howls despair; leading the dance towards the empty, hollow hopelessness that there is no point to my life.

"True" smiles delight "life is meaningless, so what's the point?" And the dance swings towards a lighter, brighter place of knowing that I, and only I, can create the point to my life.

Surrendering to survival is surrendering to the dance.

Life is meaningless and meaningful, and within that are all the reasons to kill yourself and all the reasons to live.

GARETH EDWARDS

At times despair hogs the dance so much that I want to stop dancing all together.

So instead I step off the dance floor and wait for delight to lead the dance in a different direction.

I found this happened when I learnt how to stand still.

STEP 2: STAND STILL

SURRENDERING TO SIMPLIFICATION

One of the curious things that happened once I knew I would not kill myself was the gap it left in my life.

"Should I kill myself?" had been my first thought in the morning and my last thought at night, and it would often wake me up from sleep.

It was in the background of every conversation and interaction I had with other people.

It was at the foreground of every other thought and was the lens through which I saw my problems.

GARETH EDWARDS

Work, home, relationships, money, health, happiness and my sense of purpose. I had problems with all of them. Or rather, it felt like I had one massive problem that involved all of them, that only killing myself could solve.

When that solution was delayed, I had… space.

There was space within me for different thoughts and feelings and space around me for different behaviours.

There was still a lot of 'surrendering to survival' happening.

Endless hours and days where despair dominated the dance and I relied on procrastination.

Like a parent in the supermarket being constantly asked for sweets by their child, I would often quietly reassure myself that "yes, yes dear, I will kill myself, just later darling, later".

While it felt endless at the time, it wasn't.

There were moments that became minutes, and eventually precious hours, where the child was content with the promise of sweets to come and the question of killing myself would fade.

THE PROCRASTINATOR'S GUIDE TO KILLING YOURSELF

I was a long way away from a whole day without trying to answer that question, but I was starting to get enough time to wonder what I could do instead of searching for an answer.

It was at this point that my older sister introduced me to perhaps the most valuable life skill I have ever been taught.

She called it 'standing still'.

It started with changing how I saw time.

I was approaching my 25th birthday and felt very strongly that by that point I should have my life sorted out.

Even now it is not really clear to me what having my life 'sorted out' meant.

Or even what it means now for that matter.

It seemed to involve all those things I felt I had problems with - work, home, relationships, money, health, happiness and a sense of purpose.

At the time I could only see where I was falling short of an imaginary target that I couldn't really describe beyond some sort of middle-class wet dream involving starter mortgages I didn't want and dinner parties I wouldn't want to attend let alone host.

I was losing at a game I didn't even want to play.

And worse than just losing at this game of life, I had also 'lost the plot'.

Back then I had what we used to called a 'lifestyle', which meant I took a lot of recreational drugs. And the goal seemed to be to 'lose it' on an epic LSD trip or through Ecstasy fuelled dancing.

The New Year's Eve a few weeks before my birthday I had purposefully pushed every chemical button inside my brain to see how far I could take things.

Turns out I took things too far, and by the end of News Year Day it was clear the drugs had to stop.

So I stopped.

And things got worse.

People started whispering that I had 'lost the plot'.

THE PROCRASTINATOR'S GUIDE TO KILLING YOURSELF

And whilst it was fine to 'lose it' if you were tripping or at a rave, it was definitely not fine to 'lose the plot'. That just made you a loser.

So here I was, losing at life, losing the plot and being a loser.

Not yet 25 years old I was lost and my life felt over.

Then my sister reminded me that time is something humans invented and there were two things about this that could be helpful to me.

The first was that our sense of time was something each of us set for ourselves, and it was only in our minds that something is 'taking too long' or 'going too slowly'.

So the worry that I had not 'done something with my life' was not a problem of achievement but of how I was measuring its progress towards deadlines I had absorbed from society.

More importantly, even if I was determined to 'do something with my life' (another human invention, unnecessary in my opinion), it was ok to take a little time off from the speeding treadmill my life had become.

It took a long time (or did it?) for me to accept that I wasn't failing to meet some universal checklist of 'things to do by the time you are 25'.

I still struggle with birthdays and worry that along with the birthday cards I will also get a scorecard with 'C-Minus: must try harder' or worse a straight 'F - Failed'.

But what did appeal was this idea of standing still.

Not because I was jumping for joy at the idea of stopping the relentless striving to meet goals other people and society had set for me.

Removing that particular piece of nonsense was still more than a decade away.

Standing still appealed because I had become so dysfunctional that it was impossible to strive.

I was struggling to even talk at this point and leaving the house was getting harder and harder. I was mumbling and bumbling my way through the day, hiding in my bedroom for as long as I could, thinking about killing myself.

And with little bits of time starting to come together where I wasn't thinking about killing myself I was keen to hear of any other way of existing.

Which is entirely the point.

If we can agree life is meaningless, apart from the meaning we give it, then it follows that life is just life.

That's it.

We exist.

That is the most we can really be sure of.

It is also the most we really have to do.

Just exist.

Everything else is stuff we have made up and called 'real' or stuff someone else has made up and told us is 'real'.

Take a look around you at the things that are alive.

Do you think trees are wondering what their life purpose is?

Are flowers asking each other where they see themselves in five years' time?

Do butterflies set life goals and detailed action plans to reach them?

Are monkeys taking personality tests to improve peak performance?

Do dolphins stare into the star filled night and wonder what it's all about?

Ok, maybe the dolphins do that just like we do.

But we look at nature and are happy for it to just exist, all the while forgetting that we are nature too.

Divinely designed or evolutionarily survived, we exist as part of this earth and that is it.

And sure we live in a time where it has been decided we are going to have 'jobs' and 'money', and where things like supermarkets and rent are 'real enough' that if we ignore them we will be hungry and homeless.

But our most basic requirement is to exist. To be. And when we really connect to that we can stop 'time' and stand still.

THE PROCRASTINATOR'S GUIDE TO KILLING YOURSELF

However, standing still is different from 'doing nothing'.

While our existence only requires us to be, a key part of that being is our need 'to do' - to have a useful role in our tribe or society.

We are sociable creatures and rely on connection and collaboration through doing.

So standing still is doing the least you can do without doing nothing. It is existing without purpose.

Or rather, it is existing for the purpose of existing.

It is a completely tailored, bespoke package designed to simplify your life. At the time I found it incredibly difficult and upsetting.

You might too.

First off, my sister and I set about not solving my problems. They were too big and scary, and a solution to one might make another worse.

And besides, just thinking about them made me want to kill myself.

So my sister taught me another way.

It was like creating a pause button for my problems, which meant I could let go of the pressure to fix them and also let go of the worry they might get worse if I didn't fix them.

This was so powerful for me then, and many times since, that I struggle to see how I could do anything but simplify my life when it feels overwhelming.

But back then, I felt like my career was over and I would never achieve anything.

Because of this, I would always be in debt and have to live in cheap rentals.

I'd stopped doing drugs so I thought I would lose all my friends and never make new ones.

And if I couldn't make new friends there was no chance of getting a girlfriend, which meant I would never have the family I wanted.

And my dreams of living a creative life felt completely childish and unrealistic and best forgotten.

I felt like I was giving up on life.

THE PROCRASTINATOR'S GUIDE TO KILLING YOURSELF

In a way, that was the point – to focus on 'simply living' rather than 'having a life'.

The biggest thing I simplified was my job.

I was working at a university doing a PhD and was lucky to have kind supervisors. But even then it was still difficult for me to quieten the voice telling me I was a failure and would never finish my studies.

Asking for time out was the hardest thing I had ever done in a workplace.

But in a miracle I have come to see as an everyday reality, when I clearly ask for something I really want, and it comes from a place of authenticity and good intent, I seem to get what I need. And more.

My project was put on hold and I got a job stuffing envelopes for a conference.

That might sound like a huge comedown, dropping from the heady heights of doing a PhD to be a postal clerk. And on the first day it did feel that way. I was embarrassed and ashamed and felt completely useless. But those hours in that back office became the most peaceful periods of my time learning to stand still.

I had somewhere to go and something to do that I was capable of doing.

And the amount of time where I was not dwelling on my problems or wondering if I should kill myself was growing.

This had the same effect as the procrastinating, allowing more space to kick off my tight mental shoes and let my soul toes stretch out and feel the cool breeze.

Now if this all sounds very pleasant but totally impossible for you and your work, then perhaps there is an opportunity for you to explore why that is.

For me it is usually a combination of the need to make a living and the sense of purpose my job gives me.

Having returned to this standing still approach many times I have found the more important the money is and the more responsible or well-regarded the role is, the harder it gets.

We get trapped by the lifestyle our income allows us to have and the self-importance our career gives us.

THE PROCRASTINATOR'S GUIDE TO KILLING YOURSELF

However, I also know the longer I hold off from standing still, the quicker I find myself back in despair. Just like fighting myself about wanting to kill myself makes it worse, so too does fighting myself about wanting a simpler life.

And as standing still is about doing the least I can do, the 'least' has changed as my life has changed.

For example, simplifying my work has involved sticking to my hours and not taking work home, taking less senior roles to reduce responsibilities and stepping down from management to alleviate stress.

Yes, I've also taken sick leave, quit jobs and left start-ups. And my decision to be a freelancer was partly driven by wanting flexibility in how and when I work.

None of these things were easy.

Every simplification felt complex, difficult and caused uncertainty about finances, career, vocation and my sense of purpose.

But the quicker I simplified, the less intense and lengthy those periods of despair were.

Now, if I am really quick to simplify I can skip despair almost entirely.

Standing still gave me a new way to live, allowing me to get through the days and weeks when I didn't feel I could sort out my problems.

It also gave me some solid ground on which I could step forward.

STEP 3: STEP FORWARD

SURRENDERING TO ANYTHING BUT THIS

One day I decided to go for walk.

I know that sounds unremarkable, but at the time it felt like Edmund Hillary saying 'I'm just popping out to climb Mount Everest'.

I didn't want to go for a walk.

In fact, I decidedly wanted to not go for a walk.

By this time there were only four places in the world I would go:

My doctors' surgery, to get more anti-depressants.

My counsellors' room, where I would hold back my tears for an hour.

My supervisors' office, to shake my head when asked if I was ready to return.

My local corner shop, to buy rolling tobacco and papers.

Every trip was daunting and difficult.

First I had to leave my bedroom and risk the worried smiles of my housemates who weren't sure what to say to me.

Then there was leaving the house.

The corner shop was just about do-able as I could be there and back in a few minutes.

And if I scanned the street first from the living room window, I could avoid bumping into anyone I knew.

Even then I had to prepare myself in the queue with a deep breath so that I didn't burst into tears at the till when the friendly shop owner said 'alright?'

THE PROCRASTINATOR'S GUIDE TO KILLING YOURSELF

The counsellors' room also became easier to get to, especially after the first visit where I stood on a bridge over the motorway for almost too long.

I never said much and mostly kept my British upper lip stiff while the tears gathered in my eyes.

But just to be in the presence of another person who talked gently and without judgment was profound.

The doctors' surgery was just grim. A cold, clinical reminder that I was failing as a human being and needed medical help to cope. I'm sure the people were nice, but everything they stood for made me feel like I was a crap person with a crap life.

The supervisors' office was the hardest of all. I had timed my trudge up the steep hill to the University to include an extra bit of time so I could sit down on a wall and have an intense panic attack.

Not being able to work was the surest sign I had that my life was not worth living and I was lucky the walk home did not involve bridges.

So deciding to go for a walk was a big deal.

It was my doctor who suggested that a walk might help with my depression.

That and eating more bananas.

This is what counted as 'alternative medicine' in my day.

I put on my coat and set off on a typically grey, overcast day, cupping my ever-present cigarette with my hand to protect it from the drizzle, and headed to the city's botanical park.

I had picked a week day hoping to find the park empty, but instead it was full of other sad men, clad in similar anoraks, cupping cigarettes and walking gloomily amongst the bare trees and manicured lawns.

I wondered if we all had the same doctor.

I was tempted to ask one of them if they had brought their banana.

If this was meant to be part of my treatment for 'depression', it was awfully depressing.

However, when I got home I had a small sense of achievement.

THE PROCRASTINATOR'S GUIDE TO KILLING YOURSELF

Not from going for a walk, although that did feel heroic at the time.

What impressed me was that I had done something that I had been told might help me even though I thought it wouldn't help at all.

I had tried my best.

Trying our best is the most we can ever hope to do.

Often we focus only on the goal, as if our actions are only useful if we succeed. The destination becomes 'all or nothing' and we either arrive or we fail.

I guess this is fine if we are match fit and we have a clear sense of direction.

But as I made my way back from the edge of the abyss, I had found a place where I could rest and simply 'be' for a while even though I still had no solutions to my problems or knew where my life was heading.

I was spending increasingly less time and energy thinking about killing myself, and getting into the groove of living simply and just 'being'.

In my standing still I was also starting to notice that I was able 'to do' as well as 'to be'.

As the envelope-stuffing job was coming to a finish I knew I was going to miss it.

So I started looking at what the job was giving me.

There was structure to my week, as I had to be at a certain place at a certain time. This meant I didn't have to think about what I was doing at those times.

And the task was easy enough to need a little bit of attention but without feeling stressed about whether I could do it or not. So I got to spend a little time engaged in something other than my own thoughts.

I guess it also almost meant I wasn't as useless as I felt I was. People would be getting their invitations to attend the conference and that was important for them. I was reluctant to see it this way, but I had to accept that I was kind of being useful.

Routine and doing something I was capable of doing that was of some use to someone else were the things that seemed to be bringing some relief and peace.

THE PROCRASTINATOR'S GUIDE TO
KILLING YOURSELF

So I began looking for ways to bring more of this into my life and step forward from my standing still.

I am hesitant to tell you the actual things I did because I fear you might read it like a recipe, when I feel it might be better to look at the ingredients of your life and bake your own cake.

Every thing I tried came from a place of surrender, as I really didn't want to do any of them. But I also knew that I didn't want this way of life forever.

So I surrendered to anything but 'this' – this despair, this desperate feeling that life was not worth living. If I had heard or read that something might help, I would at least try and do my best to see if it did.

I ate bananas.

I took walks.

I started cooking Sunday lunch, because it took a lot of planning and involved expeditions to the shops.

It also meant I got to spend most of Sunday washing, peeling, chopping, boiling and roasting.

GARETH EDWARDS

I seem to remember buying an old hostess trolley so I could deliver it all to my hungry housemates in the lounge.

And then I'd slope off to my room to smoke roll-ups. And eat bananas.

I decided to start watching a soap opera.

There was no TV-on-demand back then so if you wanted to watch a show you had to tune in at the time it was broadcast. That gave me three nights a week where I had an appointment of sorts.

The week after I started watching this soap opera, it began the first story about suicide ever done on TV.

It was about a young man's harrowing depression and a 'would he / wouldn't he' story line about killing himself.

I found it deeply disturbing and it was decidedly awkward for my housemates as we all watched my life mirrored on the screen in the corner of our living room.

But perhaps it was useful in an odd way, as if it were telling the story I couldn't.

THE PROCRASTINATOR'S GUIDE TO KILLING YOURSELF

Hopefully what you have noticed from these examples of my stepping forward is that none of them were about sorting out the problems I felt I had in my life. That still felt impossible and dwelling on them had me back at wanting to kill myself.

It was more like a small expansion of my standing still.

Like a king on a chessboard, I explored steps one move away from where I was.

Could I make it to the park and back? Yes.

Could I cook a nice meal for a group of people? Yes.

Could I commit to a regular TV show? Yes.

Could I eat a banana? Sure.

As my confidence grew I decided to test how far I could step forward and see if I could do something about a small but persistent problem I'd had all my life.

I joined a sign language and lip reading class.

GARETH EDWARDS

I wasn't deaf, but my hearing was poor.

I had 'ear problems' throughout childhood: grommets in two or three times a year, tonsils removed, and adenoids too. Twice.

If I got water in my ears I would lose my hearing altogether, so I never swam at school or the beach and had to have Vaseline-smeared cotton wool in my ears when I washed my hair.

One of the legacies of all this was that I struggled to hear people in groups, especially where there was lots of background noise.

I used to do a lot of grinning and head nodding in pubs and clubs and had trained myself to laugh at jokes and anecdotes when other people started laughing.

I'd always hated the impact this had on my ability to socialise, so I decided to do something about it and joined a local deaf class.

I'd say I was the youngest there by about 40 years, and the only man in the room.

It was fantastic.

THE PROCRASTINATOR'S GUIDE TO KILLING YOURSELF

The old ladies baked the sweetest cakes and didn't care what I 'did for a living'. For a few hours I wasn't a failing PhD student or a former druggie who couldn't handle it anymore.

I was just 'that nice young man who doesn't say much' and we spent a pleasant afternoon each week fiddling with our fingers and watching each other's lips move.

And it was soothing to be amongst people who didn't know me well enough to feel they had to say something to cheer me up.

While I was waiting to work out who I was, or who I could be, I was able to take a break from that pressure to present a fully formed character to the world.

I even managed to add the odd bit of cake to my banana-based diet.

The important thing about these tiny steps forward was that they were taken from a place without hope, which was still some way down the path.

I didn't believe any of these things would make my life any better. But I was willing to try.

And I think that alone meant that somewhere deep within me I did at least believe that my life could be better.

Perhaps if I tried enough things, ate enough bananas, did enough walks, created routines and things to do, gently took on some things that bothered me, then it may be possible for me to start again.

STEP 4: START AGAIN

SURRENDERING TO ENDINGS

I grew up with two sisters who loved to play dress up.

On me.

They liked to dress me up as a girl, with pigtails, freckles and rosy red lips.

Their favourite game was to lock me out of the house once they had finished and push a 10p piece through the letterbox. I was only allowed back in once I had a bag of sweets from the local shops.

One day they dressed me up as Adam Ant, with punk dreadlocks and his thick white stripe across the nose and cheeks.

The path back from the shop went alongside my local school, where in the summer the kids would hang out playing football and making mischief.

Most mischievous of all was to climb onto the roof and wait until the police arrived and then run away.

I've no idea what possessed me that day to take the detour into the school fields dressed as Adam Ant.

I think I was quite pleased with the look as he was a huge pop star at the time. I've certainly no idea why I agreed to climb up on the roof. I hated heights and had never done it before.

When the police arrived I panicked and they had to direct me to a safe place and coax me down.

There was no chance of running away.

"Name?" said the copper.

I looked at him and raised my eyebrows.

"Er… Adam?"

My pretending did not end with childhood.

I always had a sense of living two lives.

THE PROCRASTINATOR'S GUIDE TO KILLING YOURSELF

There's the one I show most of the world, of how ordinary I am.

Just a regular guy, going about his life, pursuing things like everyone else.

A solid career, steady relationship, a family, a decent house and car, some socialising at the weekend, the odd holiday somewhere sunny.

You know, a normal person.

Then there's the one I escape to when I can and that only a few people see.

The chilled-out dude, happiest strumming his guitar or aimlessly wandering around the woods. Likes to giggle and clown around, swap stories of good times and bad, and then chat until sunrise about what it's all about.

You know, a hippy.

Reconciling these two lives into a single experience is the journey of my life.

I've tried doing one or the other and so far it's proved unsatisfactory.

GARETH EDWARDS

As I approached my 25th birthday it felt like I had come to a cross roads and I had to choose one path.

The normal version of me that was doing a PhD and building an academic career felt as fake as that white stripe across my nose.

And now the fraud police had pulled me off the school roof and were asking my name!

But the hippy version of me had disappeared along with the drugs and I had yet to find a new way of playing, let alone finding new people to play with or new playgrounds to play in.

It took me many years to see it in this way, but looking back what was driving my despair was grief.

I knew my way of life – study hard, hippy harder – was over, and the prospect of all that loss was unbearable.

And with more peace and perspective arriving through surviving, standing still and stepping forward I was able to start looking at the situation I was in when the despair really started to lead the dance.

THE PROCRASTINATOR'S GUIDE TO KILLING YOURSELF

I have come to see these times where life feels unliveable as powerful signs that change is required.

I find many people struggle with this feeling that they are living somebody else's life, that it doesn't really belong to them and there is a different life waiting for them.

A happier life, with more feelings of joy and fulfilment.

It feels to me that at some point as we 'grow up' we start to push down parts of ourselves when we encounter restrictions on things we find fun.

Suddenly only some people are 'allowed' to sing or paint or make believe or run around after a ball, and they can only carry on if they take it seriously with an aim to do it 'professionally'.

And we squeeze our curiosity into little boxes marked 'school subjects' and only get rewarded when we remember bits of it and write it down in an exam hall.

Then out of nowhere, none of it actually matters anymore.

GARETH EDWARDS

We find ourselves 'grown up' and forced into this unwinnable race with no finish line, where the quality of our life is set by how many 'money' tokens we can get for doing things we would rather not do.

As we deny those parts of who we are, they start to be forgotten and replaced with the things we do to soothe ourselves in our loss.

We might take to fleeting moments of sensory pleasure in drink, drugs, food, and sex. Or we might find ways to feel like we have some power in life by buying more and more things.

Solace is found in our work, feeling important with longer hours and promotions, or trying to do jobs we feel are 'making a difference'.

And none of this is necessarily 'bad' as long as we remember that we are wild beings who belong in nature.

That our era of 'civilisation' is a new way of being we have been experimenting with for barely a few thousand years, in an existence going back hundreds of millennia.

Reality is hardly real.

THE PROCRASTINATOR'S GUIDE TO KILLING YOURSELF

When the soothing no longer soothes, our being rebels.

"No more" it says, "this must stop. I've been telling you for a long time that the path you are on is crushing your soul. This must end."

So I surrendered to the ending.

But it was not a clean surrender by any means.

Although I waved the white flag on taking drugs I'd still try them occasionally to see if anything had changed.

It hadn't.

I mourned the passing of the drug-users lifestyle: scoring, using, sorting out mates, getting high, sitting round talking nonsense, laughing until it hurt, dancing until dawn, strolling the countryside, calling in on a friend, skinning up, planning pilgrimages to Glastonbury and Amsterdam.

I missed it all and was surprised at how much time it left empty when it passed.

The hardest thing was losing my friends.

Every one of them lovely, interesting, weird, warm, funny and loving and suddenly I had walked away from our point of connection.

Even had I been able to talk, we had little left to talk about.

I wasn't expecting a miraculous return to form when I stopped taking drugs, but I was disappointed that things felt worse.

Some of it was sadness at the passing of a persona, and I'm sure some of it was a recalibrating of my brain chemicals. But what it no longer masked was that I was feeling unfulfilled by my life.

I was tired of living in cold, damp houses, racking up debt as an eternal student.

And the more academic success I had seemed to mock the creative person I longed to be but did little about.

And I wanted to love and be loved by someone I could share the journey with.

For a long time I was focused on 'fixing my problems' when it was starting to feel more like I needed to remove the source of them – my job.

THE PROCRASTINATOR'S GUIDE TO KILLING YOURSELF

It was obvious to everyone around me that I should stop doing my PhD. But I had so much of my sense of who I was wrapped up in it that it felt too big to fail. I had let my pretend life take over my whole life and put all my eggs of ambition and social approval into this one basket.

This meant surrendering was more like a war of attrition, where I chipped away at the problem until it's removal was a bit easier to swallow.

For nearly a year I toyed with ideas like redesigning the PhD project or doing it part-time. But I knew that if I returned to the same path it would lead to the same destination. It was time to stop.

I finally surrendered.

But in a way I already had.

To me 'endings' are not always as clear as they were about stopping the drugs.

A few skirmishes aside, I've not taken recreational drugs since that New Years' Day.

But even that year of exploring ways to carry on doing my PhD was an ending too, as I had decided that if I was going to continue, it would only be because I had found a new way of doing it.

So it might be that the thing at the centre of the situation that is driving the despair does not need to end entirely, just the way it's seen or being done.

But this was my first time starting again and it was the end of everything I had known until that point. After a decade of being a student and a chemical hedonist it was no longer joyful or fulfilling, so I stopped.

It meant I had to change where I lived, who I lived with, what I did for a living, and who was in my life. I had to change everything.

Since then, every return to 'starting again' has been a little less intense and dramatic. There have been some bold and audacious reboots but they have increasingly been tweaks of the situation rather than a wholesale clear out.

I think the reason for this is that I am becoming more accepting of myself.

STEP 5: SEEK SIGNIFICANCE

SURRENDERING TO SELF (OPTIONAL)

It would be easy to see this story as being about a young man who had taken too many drugs and been a student for too long, and then once he stopped messing about, his life got sorted out.

I sometimes wish that were my story.

Except it happened again. A little less intensely, but right back to wanting to kill myself and procrastinating to survive. Then having to stand still, step forward and start again.

Then it kept happening.

Over and over again I would find myself repeating

patterns of thinking, feeling and behaving and being back in similar situations. Not as dark or as bleak, and with more tools and tricks to get on with what needed to be done a little quicker and easier.

But a familiar journey, many years after the drugs and the PhD stopped.

I have come to see these as lessons of a lifetime, and that I will keep getting the same teachers until I have learnt what they have to show me about myself.

So this step is optional.

If you find 'starting again' allows you to live the life you want, that's fantastic.

But if you find you loop back to that despair again (and again) then you might want to explore the significance of this experience in your life.

The second time I found myself back wanting to kill myself I felt it was unfair. Rude even. I just wanted it to go away. I had barely got my life back and it was already under threat again.

The third time I was stunned.
It had been such a long time that I'd almost forgotten what it was like and had converted it into rampant hypochondria.

THE PROCRASTINATOR'S GUIDE TO KILLING YOURSELF

I went to the hospital emergency department convinced the panic attack I was having was a heart attack.

I didn't just do this once; I did it once or twice a week for many weeks.

And these were just the big loops, when wanting to kill myself stopped me in my tracks and demanded that I reconnect with surviving so I could stand still, step forward and start again.

There have been many more micro-loops where I have seen despair on the horizon and quickly simplified my life or skipped right to ending something so I could begin something new.

Every time I complete a spiral there is a chance to reflect on what I have learnt since the last time and be grateful that I am gathering new ideas and skills that will help this time.

And the next time.

What I am discovering is at the heart of it all is just that — a matter of the heart.

A remembering and revealing of what can be called

my 'self', the 'psyche' that is at the root of the words like psychology and psychiatry and means the human soul or spirit.

So I surrendered to myself.

I call it remembering and revealing because I believe we already know who we are.

Deep down, sometimes forgotten and painful to recall, we have a sense of self that we often hide away, shrouded in shame or embarrassment.

I am finding the more I explore and embrace that inner me, and find safe ways to take it by the hand and lead it gently towards a larger presence in my life, the more I feel whole and am better able to experience joy and fulfilment.

And the less that inner me feels like it has to stamp its feet and say, "no, this is wrong, it has to stop and if you won't stop it, I will".

The more I am truly me, the happier that me is.

But this is all looking back – High Definition, Technicolor, and Dolby surround sound hindsight.

At the time it was raw, more visceral, like a bursting feeling that if this was to be how I was going to live I had to find some way of understanding and releasing it.

I had to find meaning in the dance between despair and delight. I have seen many need to scratch a similar itch in a glorious variety of ways.

A lot of it seems to be reactivating those things we put away as we moved towards adulthood.

For me it was music and I started writing songs and eventually performing and recording them.

I've seen others find it in drawing, painting, photography, poetry, writing, singing and dancing. Others still enjoy a return to nature, walking the countryside or gardening, connecting with the earth and the wildness within.

Many find it helps to be amongst others exploring and embracing their 'self', a coming together of souls seeking significance in friendship and fellowship.
For some there is a calling to share their adventures through books, albums, talks, shows, performances. And even jobs where their personal experiences are as valued as their professional ones.

And through that sharing a new point of view is given to the world.

A unique set of ideas and perspective that someone else, perhaps someone who is soothing them self or grappling with despair, can grab hold of and draw some relief or inspiration from.

There is nothing more profound than hearing someone else speak your truth.

And when you hear that truth spoken in a way that connects to your own, you suddenly feel less alone and more empowered to move forward in your life.

If they can do it, I can do it.

If I can do it, you can do it.

ABOUT THE AUTHOUR

Gareth Edwards is a writer, entertainer and healer.

He was born in Manchester, UK (average annual hours of sunshine - 1,416) and now lives in Nelson, New Zealand (2,477. And there's a beach.)

Gareth worked in mental health for 20 years and helped design innovative services based on human rights, peer support and online self-help.

He now offers individual support to people looking for more joy and fulfilment in their life.

The Procrastinator's Guide to Killing Yourself is Gareth's first book.

For more details, visit www.gareth-edwards.com

www.ingramcontent.com/pod-product-compliance
Lightning Source LLC
Chambersburg PA
CBHW051007050726

47592CB00007B/2744